# The (delicate) art of blowjob

David Cockney

Translated from French and the
original "*L'art (délicat) de la fellation*"

# Dedication

To women of my life...

# SUMMARY

# Introduction

Did you thought to get an eyeful from reading this guide? At the risk of disappointing you, this is not an anatomy course lady. I let you the task of studying the manual and the detailed plan of the vehicle in question in this book. I'm sure most of you visualize very well the thing anyway...

This guide goes beyond the mechanical aspects of the trifle to reveal you how to give men pleasure they expect when performing the ritual dedicated to their turgid member.

This book is also not an ethics course, hygiene or sex education. Before continuing reading this, all agree that you are an adult woman wishing to improve your understanding of the thing to give more pleasure to your partner, or (and) your lovers in general.

I love and respect women too much for my words pass for vulgarity. However, I would use clear and straightforward language to describe what is to be appointed. We are after all among educated people, some intimate and well-intentioned. But dare laugh sex. Dare "clichés". Dare sharing between men and women, and for once try to understand us. Men that come from Mars, and you from nobody knows...

Finally, I ask you to believe my shared expertise on the subject of fellatio; I speak for a majority of men, including a very large majority badly sucked.

I will try to save men from industrial "Made in China" blow job by preparing future generations of suckers. This guide will allow you to access to the pantheon of snake charmers.

# Sucking is not winning

Ah, fellatio! Definitely the best time for a man to be taken by the greedy, sensual and desirous mouth of his partner.

However, if you imagine that the simple fact of doing the act offers the guarantee to fully satisfy your lover would a serious mistake. A good blowjob is not just to enjoy her partner using his mouth. This is the widest mechanics and descriptive part of the act; a common shortcut and a counterproductive approach.

In terms of oral sex, with all the respect I owe you, remember that there are many artless among you and small suck-outers. And those who claim to be the most knowledgeable often prove their perfect ignorance.

Yes, I accuse! There are some of you who, even deploying all their talents with the best will in the world remain in ignorance of what could take off the sense of man. So your ignorance makes us martyrs. My quantitative study shows that most women are deceived because of an absence or a bad practice of oral sex. To summarize: men prefer sex with women gifted to give them pleasure. After all, is it not your case beyond any other sentimental consideration?

To start, keep in mind that your body, your actions and intentions are in these moments grow your femininity to a climax. This is to flatter our ego and our pleasure.

9

I can hear the plea of the defense: "Yes but we are not always on top", "Are you kidding? We suck your dick and you are not happy?" "It gives cramps"...

Stop! My objection is clear: natural selection tends towards excellence. Life is a competition, and each individual of each species fights to access the status of good breeding. Why the hell be satisfied with mediocrity and a precarious situation while each of you has all the tools to pursue excellence and settle permanently at the top of our desires?

There are some of you very talented and others with unsuspected talents. You will find you will get amazing results with less effort by following my tips.

# Setting the Stage

For starters, there's really no established rule. Depending on the degree of your partner's excitation and the blowjob's context that can sometimes be practiced quickly in a park or a carriage driveway, you will provide the care to your man cock at more or less advanced stages. If instead you have all the time: take it!

An extreme excitement is the key to a successful introduction. Like you, is not it ladies? Also, I would strongly advise you to turn around the beast and titillate before introducing it in your mouth. Because the envy you complete the job and the representation we do actually participate in a large part to the pleasure of this gratification. This can be accentuated using speech during your actions.

Caress his hypothalamus before his diabolical device so that your mouth craves. I'm not talking about masturbation at this stage. There must be a contact. First light, then more accentuated. For starters, you can step through his pant or boxer (yes, shorts and underpants are outdated, tell him ...).

When his sex is amply rigid and begins to look at you with pleading, by contracting, moving the pelvis, rubbing your hair ... continue to undress slowly.

I would strongly recommend you to contemplate his sex but caressing everywhere else (preferably) before interest you to his penis.

You can then start to kiss gently around sex (without too much with your hair or tickle your nose in the hollow of the groin). The secret of this perioral step is important: take your time and let your partner anticipate. This will make his desire grow. This should produce in him a surge of desire that will do for much of the "work".

Then turn around his cock, caressing the tip of the finger from the bottom up and top down. Kiss it over the entire length and testes. Pull slowly his penis very gently rubbing the crown of the latter with the pads of your fingers.

Make him feel your breath, and the tip of your tongue on his skin ... a little moan ... a pinch lips, envious and greedy eyes ... Lengthen this stage a few moments always adding more gluttony (more lips and more tongue). This is actually a crescendo, essential to any good symphony. If you do not neglect this pre-oral step, he should pray that you take it soon in your delicate mouth.

You must reach a natural lubrication of his sex by its pre-seminal fluid. Just as your love juice, this lubrication is a good indication of his state of excitement. If it is not obvious or if you do not have signs of agitation, even more slowly continue without focusing on his penis.

Start into your ritual hugs on the bit of the tip of your tongue supported by alternating stimuli. For uncircumcised, remove his foreskin in a back-and-coming, then take hold of its tail very slowly by touching his entire penis with your fingers. The crown of the glans is very sensitive and stimulating at a great excitement causes shivers of excitement.

Continue this step by varying the pleasures of kisses, delicate strokes of tongue, becoming longer and targeted leads until the edge of his enjoyment.

When you feel lubrication and excitement, take it gently in the mouth, slowly.

Start up to half of the glans very slowly so he can enjoy (and you too), the warmth of your lips, the moisture from your mouth and finally feel the slight movements of your tongue...

Return to the charge, alternately pause and appetizers increasingly the strength of your movements. It is not necessary to unroll the entire cable violently early or shaking it like a savage.

Keep a reserve for the end ... Play of his enchanted flute crescendo. I repeat myself? Go GRADUALLY.

David Cockney

# Main course

He is on the verge of enjoyment; you got him entirely in your mouth and feel the edge of explosion? It's time to get out your perverse arsenal.

The party should just begin at this point. Calm down a little your manual stimulation to not to enjoy him too fast.

No need to open your mouth, pretending you want to collect his sperm immediately in the manner of a porn star. This will excite him for sure, but if it is too early for him, he could think that you are already tired, which is likely to spoil his party.

Do not terminate the game in the first half. What's the secret of a good blowjob? A total purge! You must empty his testicles which should ultimately look like a tea bag drained. Stuck for inspiration to go slowly?

Nibble his foreskin delicately, style your hairs; in short: make some diversion. Abrupt withdrawal, the unexpected slowdowns or rhythm delay the coming of ejaculation.

Important point: make sure that the phallus your man is always properly lubricated with saliva. Especially his penis, that is very sensitive to frictions and irritations. No need either of us play porn star spitting violently on it.

You will not beat records with nets or drooling, shaking him violently. Subtly salivate. Your technique should be delicate hairlines and your gestures, in a demonstration of gluttony and sensuality.

Show your man you love what you do will make 75% of the work. Much of his fun is going on in his proper head.

The fact that you are attracted to him and devoted her gender is a key to his pleasure.

So you need to show you nasty and greedy, and avoid forcing you.

Because there is nothing more unpleasant for a man to see his disgusted partner or irritated impatience.

So you must make him feel that you love what you do. Smell his sex, eat it greedily, look at him with envy, take deep breaths, howl and regularly carry a strong look at your partner.

You must subtly alternate the manual and oral stimulation by varying the pressure and without insisting more than 30 seconds in a raw to a single technique.

Men love surprises and changes of speed. In addition, a change will rest your maxillaries... Do not hesitate to lick the entire length and testicles between some back and forth. You must alternate the targeted areas and then to swallow greedily again and again.

Glans ring is the most sensitive part of him, but the heat to be taken entirely will melt him of pleasure. Gently grab his testicles also.

Many women wonder if men would rather be swallowed entirely in the throat. The answer is yes!

Not during the whole act, but at least from time to time and especially at the end. However, this should not be too forced to wring risk sex and above to make you vomit.

You must know your limits, but try to increase by practicing a simple sword swallower technique.

You know that sinking something in your throat causes the vomiting reflex. To avoid this natural protective reflex, it is quite possible to act by swallowing to counteract it and clear the way to your partner's penis.

To gain a few centimeters, you can also put you on the back or in "69" position to allow deeper penetrations in your mouth.

Remember to gently guide him if he goes too far (and he will be tempted to go, trust me).

Come now deep gorges that will please your man ... I'm almost jealous.

David Cockney

# It could spoil the party...

Before tackling the grand finale of your explosive fireworks, let me highlight a few important points that could be qualified as negligence.

**The "kneading the crank" mode.** Some of you often shake our penis violently, probably expecting efficiency. Sometimes it works. But I arrest you right now: even the hottest loose valuable credits when they leave the milking machine in automatic mode. In addition, it is much more tiring for you.

**Pulling too hard on his testicles.** Never forget that they are connected by veins and sperm ducts in the abdomen. Their stretching causes very unpleasant pain and that persist long moments. Sucking not bite or snatch her jewel, even if you love to play with...

**Play piano on her sex for fun.** This is definitely NOT fun. There is nothing more annoying than seeing his partner to take this action with detachment. It will make you laugh alone.

**Go tight-lipped.** I cannot count the number of girls practicing fellatio, pursing lips or covering their teeth with. No !

Fellatio is a perilous exercise, but you should reduce the risk of injury by your delicacy, and not some ridiculous ruse that annihilates all forms of pleasure. I will not repeat it anymore: you should suck your partner with the fleshiest hottest and wettest parts of your mouth! No lip. You are a femme fatale, not a saint minx.

**Snorkeling.** I practice this sport and, believe me, there's little chance you get to hold more than a minute, waving on the sex of your partner.

It's frustrating for him and difficult for you. Especially if your partner is not a premature ejaculator, you may syncope. This is why you must breathe with the nose alternating techniques and sometimes open your mouth a little bigger to have good inspirations.

A blowjob is not an endurance or speed contest anyway. Keeping constantly his sex in your mouth is not as pleasant for him, but for you the guarantee of jaw cramps.

**Getting upset.** There is nothing less exciting for him; it's very annoying. Please control your nerves, even though being a pain in the ass is in your genes. This is not the moment to warm up an old argument.

At this time the star it's him. Just focus on his pleasure. He will certainly give back your attentions on another occasion; making you enjoy, giving you a ring, flowers or by any act of romance as McDonalds invitation or refraining him from farting.

If at any time you are in an uncomfortable position (he pulls your hair, press your head), know that the excitement causes impulses and it is only the effect of his excitement; this is proof of your talent.

Try to be diplomatic in all circumstances.

Take note of his advanced excitement and just guide his gestures with tact.

**Talking with your mouth full.** I would not allow myself this notice if it was not necessary and if the chitchat was not so common among women.

Please, ladies, this time is certainly not the time to tell your working day or plan your weekend.

This is not because we do not like you, but simply because it is not currently. A good blow job is done in silence. Did you say "macho"? Men simply operate like that.

We know only do one thing at a time and our minds are focused on your mouth and pleasure it gives.

Yes, men know how to give up completely and not think about anything other than sex. Besides, if we happened to think of something else, we would know.

The only words that should get out of your mouth at this moment are about "I love your cock", "I love to suck you" and "come in my mouth."

Practice self-censorship and strict filtering on your words and you'll get good results.

To sum up: to show signs of impatience, pause, blow effort or report that he is long playoffs are on the way to the royal grail pipe.

If you are tired or if he is unusually long, it is simply that you did wrong or have neglected foreplay.

To become more effective, use your complicity to make him say what he likes most and least to become his sucker of record.

You know very well ask ourselves about where we are when we put too much for 30 minutes home from work. So why not leverage your Gestapo agent's talent to try to guess our desires?

**Blow or lick his urethra.** Ouch! The urethra is a direct opening on the inner lining of his sex.

They are very sensitive and irritable. To summarize this pique violently and slip your tongue would be a grave wrong note in your symphony.

Finally, if you get to this point by having foiled the main obstacles to the dream blow job, you are on the path of extreme pleasure and to your partner gratitude. You finally will get the power to hold men by the intimacy of their origins.

# Expert's surprises

Here before achieving your work, some tricks or tips to experiment that can heighten your partner's pleasure...

## *The warm feather*

During preliminary to oral introduction, barely touching the brake and his penis with the tip of your tongue without further contact that it should make him mad.

If you are quite distant at first then very gradually concentrated on his penis, he should quickly beg that you take him in your mouth.

To the cinema, in the dark, with the pressure of the environment, this practice should make sparks when he expects a quick treat. And even if you do not go after, be sure to see his excitement at work on the way back.

## *Gluttony*

If you start around champagne accompanied with sushi, avoid sucking him with champagne or wasabi.

However, honey, Nutella and whipped cream are great allies to show your appetite. Remember: be creative, and gourmet!

## Norwegian pipe

Blow hot and cold using fresh stuff. Brush your teeth with minty toothpaste or just suck an ice while you practice your art. The sensations of your partner are guaranteed!

## Put him under pressure

As the stimulation comes and goes in your mouth to simulate penetration and action of its basin in privacy, vary the pressure to simulate sometimes caresses, sometimes close penetration. You can occasionally exaggerate the pressure on his penis to feel the contractions and see it swell with desire.

## The washer

While sucking, do a circle between your thumb and your index finger to masturbate him. By exercising some pressure to maintain his excitement it will simulate a narrow penetration as sodomy. Furthermore, if you masturbate while you suck stimulates greater zone as a deep gorge.

## Prostate madness

If this idea disgusts you, skip this paragraph. I want to warn you; all men do not like this practice.

Either because they are psychologically refractory because of their education, either because they are not very receptive.

However, I can bet my money that there are a lot of men who love the pressure of a well-placed finger in their anus to stimulate their prostate just before the end of the act.

If your complicity is big enough with your partner you could test the waters starting with some pressure from his scrotum to his hole.

The idea to sodomize their man excites some women. If this is the case and he likes it, just do it!

David Cockney

# Then comes dessert

You have already done much of the way at this stage and avoided the major pitfalls. The dish should be widely consumed and your partner at the extreme edge of enjoyment. He turned a corner of no return and it is time to achieve the menu.

With time and your certainty of his excitement, you will soon become the queen to anticipate the moment of his ejaculation.

Take time to discover the tastes of your partner and be attentive to his reactions. More you practice more you will concentrate your efforts on the things that work on him.

If you want to do enjoy, you now just have to further accelerate your pace and show you ready to collect his manhood.

Your greedy gaze and your subtle moans should suggest him to honor your mouth, your breasts, your face, your chest...

No man should force his wife to swallow his ejaculate with relish.

If your partner's sperm is something repugnant to you, so do not plan to swallow. But suggest it will increase his pleasure greatly.

For more reluctant, sperm is all that is healthy if your

partner is too. It takes its source in a sterile environment.

Moreover, it is not at all caloric (about 30 Kcal per ejaculation) and is no more disgusting that some of your herbal tea or diet drinks.

Anyway, you need at this stage to show him that you are having fun and suggest you are gourmand. All men want to sprinkle the face, mouth or chest of their partner by ejaculating. If you suggest that you are ready for it, you will significantly increase his pleasure at the top of his enjoyment.

The first sperm spurts should not be an issue for you and certainly no sign of stopping abruptly.

You should instead prolong his pleasure to lead him to total relaxation.

Masturbate your partner a little more gently.

Take it in the mouth moments, caress it, lick it ... and kiss him.

Wait a few moments before looking for a handkerchief or run to the bathroom.

The hardening of her nipples, the contraction of his balls, his sighs, his skin, his touch, his kisses and his eyes should thank you.

If you succeed, he will want to retain you for a long time...

# Conclusion

The discovery of your partner's meaning and pleasure in the practice of oral sex are large and infinitely rich.

My final tip is to take pleasure in what you do, without forcing you.

Be attentive to the direction of your lover and conscious mechanisms of male pleasure.

Finally find a partner with whom you'll want to give this pleasure and give you up entirely.

The best things are made with envy.

If you want to share with me your experience or suggestions to improve this work, you can write me at david.cockney@gmail.com.

Now I'm jealous of the guy who will be the next in your expert hands.

Stop joking. Thanks for reading this book.

With my affection and friendship...


David

David Cockney

www.ingramcontent.com/pod-product-compliance
Lightning Source LLC
Chambersburg PA
CBHW061945280526
45787CB00004B/1731